By the same author:

The Great Big Anthology of Laughter Exercises
Laughter Revolutionaries: Making the World Safe for
Hilarity (available in Italian translation)
Froigen deebled Craggle-zorp! : The All-Gibberish Photo-
and Story-book
Moving Experiences : A Manual for Awakening (with
Ruthe Gluckson)
The Laughter Club in Real Time (DVD)
Gibberish Sets You Free! – Five short films on the power
of talking nonsense (DVD)
Gibberish Kit (with Dr. Madan Kataria) (four-DVD set)
Laughter Exercise Photo Flash Cards
Come to the Laughter Club (MusicVideo)
The Laughalong March (MusicVideo)
The Ho Ho Ha Ha Laughter March (Music Video)

The author moderates a laughter lovers' online support
group, "Laugh4Health" at YahooGroups.com

The Laughter Yoga Book

Laugh Yourself to Better Health

Physical ~ Mental ~ Emotional
Social ~ Spiritual

Jeffrey Briar

The Laughter Yoga Book (Compact Edition)

© 2016 The Laughter Yoga Institute

ISBN-13: 978-1478292135

ISBN-10: 147829213X

Creative Arts Press
790 Manzanita Drive
Laguna Beach, California USA

Note to the reader: This book is intended as an informational resource. The techniques described herein are not meant to substitute for professional medical care or treatment. Consult with your healthcare professional before engaging in any physically demanding activity or making any changes in your treatment program.

What's Inside

Laughter Buddies

Doctor Madan Kataria and Jeffrey Briar

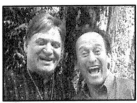 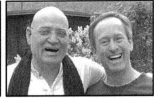

May, 2005 ~~~ May, 2011

Wilderswil, Switzerland

Forward by Dr. Madan Kataria

It gives me great pleasure to present Jeffrey Briar's book, which will prove to be a great resource for anyone who wants to bring more laughter into their life, and also if they want to help others to have more laughter in their lives.

Laughter Yoga is a unique, reliable system to deliver the health benefits of hilarity. This technique allows everyone to laugh, whether you have a sense of humor or not; whether you are happy or you are not happy.

The idea is simple. You don't need any kind of mat or shoes, you just get together in a group and laugh. Its uniqueness lies in its unconditional, common language: everyone speaks "Ha ha ha!" You don't need any language mechanism to understand. Humor needs the language mechanicals, but Laughter Yoga is unconditional. Laughter Yoga works better than humor to provide sustained laughter. Laughter Yoga is unconditional. People only need to know that laughing without a reason, without jokes – this laughter is effective. Now we have proven this.

We are not against humor. We just don't need to rely on it in order to laugh. **Laughter is too important to be dependent on jokes.** If you laugh a few seconds here or there throughout the day that does not alter your physiology significantly. By doing laughter as an exercise, we can laugh for fifteen or twenty minutes, and that *will* bring about physiological changes.

Laughter Yoga began with only five people. Now there are hundreds of thousands of people practicing Laughter Yoga all over the world. One reason for this incredible growth is that Laughter Yoga was introduced in a public park. Health-conscious people were already there, doing group activities. Those who came for a walk got the added benefits of laughter, and those who came for laughter got walking - double the benefits. Once experienced, it became self-sustaining.

Another reason for the phenomenal growth is that Laughter Clubs are free of cost, and thus available to everyone. Many people want to do health-building activities, but there can be some resistance if they have to pay for it. In India things which are free of cost are nonetheless perceived as having potential value. Thus people could easily experience that laughter as exercise was good.

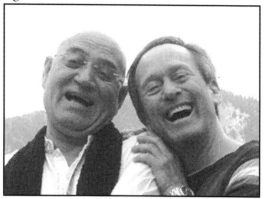

Dr. Kataria and the Author

In fulfillment of our mission to spread good health, happiness and joy, we are creating The International Laughter Yoga University, a university which does not offer academic degrees but will instead teach people how to have more laughter in their lives. The University will have four divisions: Singing, Dancing, Playing, and Laughing. There will be a Center for Holistic Healing and Integrated Medicine; departments of Yogic Science and Ayurveda, Acupuncture, and even Laughter Spirituality. Laughter Tours and Holidays will organize group sightseeing tours which emphasize "fun as you learn".

One of the major objectives of the university is to conduct scientific research on the healing effects of Laughter Yoga and other alternative health systems.

The university will have a full-fledged Department of Joy, and when we open the Division of Gibberish, there is a fellow I have in mind to keep everyone laughing.

Jeffrey Briar has been associated with the Laughter Yoga movement ever since its inception in the United States. He has been instrumental in spreading the laughter movement. He was the first to start a free seven-days-per-week laughter club in the western world.

What impresses me is not just his knowledge about Laughter Yoga, but his passion for bringing laughter into the lives of many people.

Being a teacher of traditional Yoga is also a valuable addition to blend with Jeffrey's knowledge of and experience with Laughter Yoga.

I am confident that you will get great value and insight from enjoying Jeffrey's book.

(Portions excerpted with permission from an interview published in *Laughter Revolutionaries: Making the World Safe for Hilarity* from the present author; and from *Laugh for no Reason* by Madan Kataria, MD)

Introduction

Laughter as Exercise

Can you laugh even if you don't feel like it, even if you don't find anything funny?

It's often said that "Laughter is the Best Medicine" but how can you get a healthy dose when you need it, even if you are in a bad mood or there's nothing to laugh at?

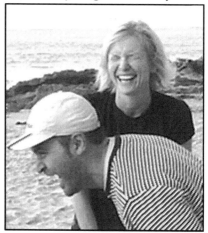

This book will show you how.

You *can* have an abundance of laughter in your life, on demand, whenever you want.

Laughter Yoga is a technique of producing laughter for its own sake, without needing jokes or comedy. Participants interrelate playfully like children having fun together at a playground. Thanks to the social interaction, the laughter quickly becomes genuine and heartfelt.

Laughter Yoga was created in 1995 by Dr. Madan Kataria, a physician in India, in collaboration with his wife Madhuri, a yoga teacher. It began with five people in a park in Bombay. Hundreds of thousands of people worldwide now practice laughter for health.

A typical laughter session includes: Easy stretches, breathing practices, and an assortment of laughter techniques, such as those you will find in this book. The exercises are simple and very pleasant to perform. There is no need for costly equipment, mats, or special clothing. Participants choose their level of involvement, from gentle to vigorous; the experience is suitable for all ages and all levels of ability. Laughing classmates tend to form caring, supportive friendships. Participants live life more joyfully, and find themselves better able to cope with whatever stresses life may bring.

Why Laugh?

In the 1960's, journalist Norman Cousins (see pp. 50-53) cured himself of a painful disease diagnosed terminal through the use of alternative therapies which included watching a steady supply of funny laughter-invoking movies and TV shows. His book *Anatomy of an Illness* led to extensive medical research.

Benefits of Laughter may include:

- Relieves stress - reduces adrenaline and cortisol
- Lessens anxiety, fear, depression - raises serotonin levels
- Enhances the immune system - boosts natural anti-viral and anti-cancer cell activity
- Improves respiratory and cardiovascular systems - dilates blood vessels, normalizes blood pressure; increases lung capacity, increases oxygen levels in the blood and the brain
- Relieves pain - produces an endorphin-like effect
- Encourages relaxation of muscles and mind
- Boosts self-confidence, promotes compassion, deepens creativity

To achieve significant health effects, laughter needs to be of sufficient duration. An occasional chuckle is a good practice but does not lead to the desired results. Most studies declare ten to twenty minutes as the Recommended Allowance to achieve these physiological benefits. Jokes and comedy are not reliable sources for generating laughter lasting such a length of time, but Laughter as Exercise can dependably do the job.

Thanks to the discovery and development of this kind of Laughter without Jokes, *you need never remain stressed-out again.*

Laughter for your Life

Laughter activities make practical and popular additions to yoga classes, at senior center activities, and for business meetings. When you attend sessions with laughter you are more likely to enjoy the class, be less self-critical, and develop more friendships. You can anticipate feeling less pain and that your mood will be happier and more outgoing.

Teachers of laughter-infused classes find that overall class attendance goes up. Laughter "breaks" during meetings and study sessions result in more focused attention, better retention and greater involvement. Laughter in the workplace leads to employees who are genuinely happy to go to work every day.

Laughter evoked from playfulness and fun has the same benefits as laughing at a joke - laughing "at" something perceived as funny. We *can* laugh deliberately, as an expression of lightheartedness and joy; we don't need to first judge something as humorous or amusing.

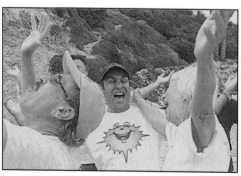

**Laughing while having fun
is just as good as laughing at something funny**

Welcome to the World of Unconditional Hilarity

Laughter Yoga presents a revolutionary new concept: Laughter as Exercise.

Using this breakthrough technique, *anyone* can laugh, abundantly and for a prolonged period of time. There is no need for jokes, comedy, or even having a sense of humor. Everyone can laugh, even if they are feeling sad, anxious, or bored.

Laughing encourages the sense of humor. Laughter itself, performed with a playful and childlike attitude, generates the Chemistry of Happiness.

Psychologists say that one of the tragedies of depression is that depressed people cannot laugh. They go on to say that people who laugh frequently don't seem to get depressed. This book encourages everyone to laugh regularly as a form of preventive medicine, so that none of us need ever fall into a state of depression.

Where can you find Unlimited Free Laughter?

Laughter Yoga is a global phenomenon. It started in India in 1995 with a small group – only five people. At the time of this writing (2016) there are an estimated 10,000 laughter clubs in 90 countries; 350,000 people all over the world laugh regularly as a form of exercise to improve their health.

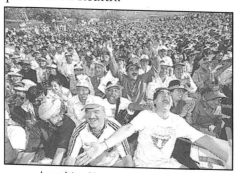

Laughter Yoga session in India

What is "laughter" – What happens when we laugh?

Laughter involves breathing, vocalization, and contractions (and release) of the epiglottis of the throat. We inhale a quantity of air, and then expel that air, which passes over the vocal chords to create the sounds of laughter. The thoracic diaphragm is engaged to activate the lungs. While laughing, blood vessels dilate, allowing for an easier flow of blood through the vascular system. This has a beneficial effect on the function of the heart. Blood pressure tends to normalize as the result of regular laughter practice.

Laughter assists the flow of lymph through the body's lymphatic system. Lymph has an important function in cleansing our bloodstream from waste products and unwanted invaders. However, the lymphatic system does not have a muscle to push the lymph (while the vascular system has the heart muscle to pump the blood through the circulatory system). We need to engage in physical movement in order to move lymph. Lymph can also be moved through laughing. Such vigorous internal movement also aids the functioning of the systems of digestion and elimination.

Try it Yourself: Laugh Right Now for No Good Reason (No Jokes)

Here's an easy-to-perform experiment whereby you can feel the immediate benefits of deeper breathing and intentional laughter.

Sit comfortably in a chair with space in front of you such that you will be able to lift your arms forward and up above your head. (You can stand, if you prefer.) Have both feet flat on the floor and your back straight. Take an inhalation through the nose while lifting your arms above your head. Take in as large a breath as possible and hold your arms up for a good stretch. Then slowly lower the arms back 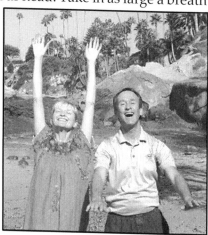 towards your waist while breathing out through the mouth. Put extra emphasis on the exhalation in a gentle effort to empty the lungs of all remaining air.

Repeat this deep inhalation while raising the arms, and deep exhalation while lowering them, three more times. Now close your eyes and check in with yourself: "How do I feel? Tired, or energetic? If rating myself in 'feeling good', on a scale from 1 to 10, where am I? Down at 2 or 3, or up at 8 or 9?"

Now let's try it with laughter.

Still with the feet flat and the back straight, take a big breath in while raising the arms up. This time, as you lower the arms, make sounds of laughter. It doesn't matter if the laughter seems forced or artificial; we are doing an experiment to see how breathing with sound - in this case, laughter sounds - might effect the way we feel. Make sounds like "Ha ha ha," "ho ho ho," "hee hee hee" or any combination.

Repeat this practice of inhaling deeply while the arms are lifted, then laughing deeply while lowering the arms, four times.

Now pause and close the eyes. Check in again: "How do I feel? What is my energy level? How do I feel emotionally? If I rated myself in 'feeling good' on a scale from 1 to 10..."

Most people find that the practice of a few breaths with laughter boosts their mood and improves their energy level. Some feel more alert and refreshed; others feel a sense of relaxation and calm. Whatever you feel or don't feel is fine. Even simply taking some deep breaths is going to be beneficial to your respiratory system. When we add laughing, we increase the number and range of health benefits.

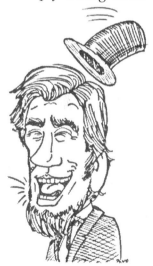

"With the fearful strain that is upon me night and day, if I did not laugh, I should die. " – Abraham Lincoln

21

Laughter Undoes the Damaging Effects of *Stress*

Perhaps the number one benefit of laughter is that it neutralizes the negative effects of physical and emotional stress.

"Stress" is a term which has been borrowed from the fields of physics and architecture. To an architect, stress is "-a force acting upon a structure against which the structure must compensate or lose its structural integrity.-" If you build a floor on the fifth story of a building, anticipating that anticipate *people* will be walking on that floor, you need that the floor and walls will have a certain structural strength. However, if you anticipate hordes of *elephants* will be walking on that same floor, the floor and the walls will need to be made with much stronger materials and supports. Otherwise, the greater weight of the elephants - a much greater "force" creating a much higher degree of "structural stress" - may result in the collapse of the floor or walls of the building.

In the 1920s, research scientist Hans Selye (p. 49) began using the term "stress" to describe physical and emotional challenges placed on human beings. We now use the term to indicate the reaction to a perceived life-threatening emergency; the Fight-or-Flight or Alarm Response.

When we perceive something as a danger to our survival, we go into a state of heightened anxiety. The adrenal glands located atop the kidneys release powerful compounds called catecholamines into our bloodstream. Adrenaline and cortisol cause a rise in our blood pressure, to send blood to the large muscles - legs, arms - to run away from (flee) or fight off the attacker. At the same time, our blood vessels constrict, so if we are wounded by the offensive beast, blood loss will be minimal. However, constricted blood vessels also result in reduced blood flow to the brain. We can't think well when we are stressed.

In the Stress/Alarm Response our breathing gets shallow; we are ready to make a quick dash away from the danger. The immune, digestive, and reproductive systems effectively shut down. Our body wants us to *get out of there* – to run away from the danger. Only later, *if* we survive, can we focus on deeper relaxed breathing, a calm heart, eating, and thinking clearly again.

Stress Surrounds Us

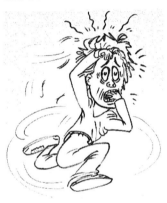

The problem is that in our modern life, stressors are everywhere, and occur nearly all of the time. High-pitched traffic noises will give us the stress response, as will sudden bright lights. We can even thrust ourselves into the Fight-or-Flight response by having upsetting thoughts (e.g.: "What if something bad were to happen?").

Fortunately, **laughter undoes the negative effects of stress**. As a result of laughing: blood vessels dilate, breathing deepens; stress factors like adrenaline and cortisol dissipate. After laughing: relaxation follows, blood pressure normalizes; we can eat and think more comfortably.

Benefits the Immune System

Several researchers have shown that laughter can improve the functioning of the immune system. This system gives us protection against harmful and invasive substances such as bacteria, viruses, and cancer. Research by Dr. Lee Berk (p. 53) suggests that laughter may increase production of lymphocytes, Immunoglobulins, and Gamma Interferon. Berk's research also showed that natural anti-cancer cell activity is up-regulated as a result of mirthful laughter.

Good for the Heart, Blood and Brain

Research by Dr. Michael Miller showed that laughter has a direct effect on the blood vessels.   Subjects in this study showed constriction (closing) of their blood vessels when they watched a frightening film, but dilation (opening) of the blood vessels when they laughed at a comedy movie. A better flow of blood (improved "systemic pressure") means it is easier for the heart to do its job of pumping the blood through the vascular system. Thus laughter might be said to help regulate blood pressure. This improved blood flow can effect the entire system, including the brain. Better flow of blood to the brain means better brain function and better thinking.

Breath is Life

When we laugh, we actively expel air from the lungs. Thus we will evacuate old, stale air along with carbon dioxide and other waste gases. After we blow the old air out, we bring fresh air in, thereby increasing oxygen levels in the lungs and on into the bloodstream.

The Thoracic Diaphragm is a muscle often described as mushroom- or parachute-shaped.

It attaches to the sternum in the front of the rib cage and to the spine in back. It can be said to separate the hard, bony rib cage from the soft, 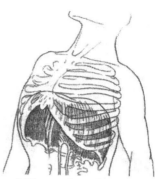 vulnerable abdomen. When the diaphragm descends towards the pelvis, the lungs expand downward, drawing in fresh air. When the diaphragm moves up towards the throat, the lungs are compressed, pushing out the air in the lungs. When we laugh, the diaphragm moves rapidly up and down. This action gives a gentle massage to our inner organs, including the heart - the kind of massage which helps these organs function at their best.

The typical human Lung has a total capacity of about 6000 milliliters (~ 1.6 gallons). If you could expand your lungs and draw in every possible molecule of air, there could be 6000 mL of air within those lungs.

If you could push out as much air as possible, there still would remain a certain volume. This is called the Residual Volume, and represents 1500 mL (~ 1.6 quarts). This means the amount of air which *can* be drawn into the lungs (called the Vital Capacity) is 4500 mL (4.5 liters, or ~1.2 gallons).

A typical breath pushes out, and then

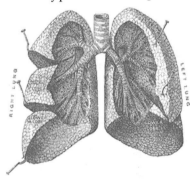

brings in, only 500 mL of air – about two cups. That's all. We breathe in only two cups of air, when we have the *potential* to breathe in 1.2 *gallons* – nine times that amount. By the act of deliberately laughing, we can hope to push out (and then bring in) 1500 to 2500 mL of air. We can increase our intake of air by a factor of 3 to 5 times. More air in means more oxygen in., and since laughter causes the blood to be transported more effectively throughout the body, we may have higher levels of oxygen in the blood and brain. This can result in feeling more energetic and thinking more clearly.

Digestion and Elimination

Research scientist William Fry (p.54) described laughter as "Internal Jogging". Laughter could be considered a form of mild aerobic exercise with similar benefits for breathing as well as improving the digestive and eliminative systems. Laughter can help us to eliminate wastes through both the digestive and lymphatic system, as mentioned earlier.

Pain Relief

Dr. Fry also said that laughter causes the release of endorphins, the body's natural painkillers.

The ability of laughter to relieve pain was also noted by journalist Norman Cousins (see quote p. 52). People who attend laughter sessions often cite the alleviation of pain as one of the favorite results from their laughter practice.   Later we will discuss the effect of endorphins on emotional well-being.

Living a Pain-Free Life

There are other fitness programs which use the slogan "No Pain, No Gain." Laughter Yoga does not subscribe to that theory. With Laughter Yoga, feeling good is fundamental. Laughter has proven pain-relieving effects, but we don't want to take advantage of that to over-exert or over-stretch ourselves.

The primary consideration is expressed in the imperatives "No New Pain" and "Take Good Care of Yourself."   Laughter Yoga participants only want to feel good, or better, at the end of the session as well as afterwards. Any laughter exercise, movement or stretch which might cause pain or discomfort can be avoided. Every activity can be modified to fit the comfort level of the participant. If a laugher begins to feel faint or nauseous, they can discontinue the exercise, relax and breathe comfortably.

What do 'Sex, Drugs, and Rock-and-Roll' have in common with Laughter?*

[*The author sends special thanks to Dr. Michaela Schaefner for using this catchy title in a Laughter Yoga presentation she gave to a conference of Rolfing therapists in Germany.]

Many things bring pleasure. Massage and soothing touch, chocolate and "comfort foods", rhythmic music and other stimulants cause an increase, in certain areas of the brain, of the neurotransmitter *Dopamine*.

(Dr. Lee Berk and Dr. Earl Henslin, at the 2012 conference of the Association for Applied and Therapeutic Humor, came up with the following neuro-pharmacological answer to the question "What is happiness?" "**Happiness is Dopaminergic up-regulation in the Nucleus Accumbens of the brain**.") ('Kind of takes the romance out of it, doesn't it?)

A neurotransmitter is a substance which supports the transmission of energy along neuronal pathways (conduits of energy-information in the brain). When we have an abundance of Dopamine in a specific area of the brain (the Nucleus Accumbens) we get the

message: "That feels good – keep doing that."
It's part of a biofeedback mechanism which
rewards us for doing behaviors which
contribute to our well-being. Dopamine levels
go up (we feel "good") when we give and
receive affection, when we are being kind to
others, and when receiving the kind attention
of others. We get similar positive brain
chemistry-feedback from eating foods which
support our survival.

Some substances cause high concentrations
of Dopamine in the pleasure/reward center of
the brain. Cocaine can increase concentrations
of Dopamine as much as 500 times. Such
substances - cocaine, heroin, alcohol, etc. - can
prove extremely addictive. We want the
pleasure we feel from the substance without
consideration for the cost. Addiction to such
substances can lead to diminished social
function, with negative behaviors ranging
from lack of caring for others to acts of crime.

Laughter may increase Dopamine
concentrations as high as fifty times, but it does

not seem to have any negative side effects. (No one is likely to break into your car and steal your stereo in order to buy a DVD of *Seinfeld* reruns.) Laughter could be said to be a positive addiction, as are aerobic exercise, eating nourishing foods, and performing acts of kindness. It might be more accurate to describe such actions not as "addictions" but rather as "healthy habits".

Simply put: ***Laughter creates the Chemistry of Happiness.***

When a person laughs abundantly they do not feel stressed nor anxious. People who laugh often tend to not get depressed. Reliable, pleasurable brain chemistry can result in people feeling more confident and having better self-esteem. The deliberate practice of laughter also develops a person's sense of humor – their ability to laugh at whatever life brings. This softening of the attitudes will in itself result in diminished levels of emotional stress.

Varieties of Laughter Exercises

Laughter Yoga exercises can be divided into three types.

Category 1: From Traditional *Hatha Yoga*

Yogic breathing techniques (*Pranayama*) and postures (*Asanas*) adapted for use as laughter practices.

Namaste Greeting

Instruction: "Place the palms of the hands together in front of your heart. Go up to

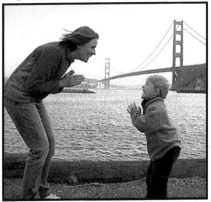

another person, bow slightly, keeping eye contact. Laugh with their Inner Child.

(Yours, too!) Mingle around and repeat with many others."

Lion Laughter

"Stick your tongue way out and down towards the chin; make a big smile; lift the eyebrows high, with eyes open wide; put the hands

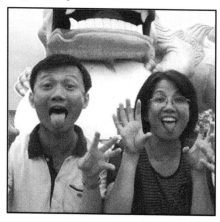

to the sides of the face shaped like a lion's paws (fingers up); roar laughter deep from your belly. Be 'frightened' by the other lions. Then, pounce back!"

Salutation to the Fun

"Interlace your fingers below the waist, palms towards the belly. Inhaling, bring the hands towards your face, then the arms up, palms to the sky. Exhaling, separate the hands, lower the arms down by the thighs."

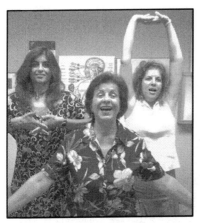

To add Laughter: "Stretch the arms up and hold, breath in; when you can't hold the breath any longer, burst out laughing as you release the hands. You can move around, interact; return the arms up and lower as desired.

Category 2: Playful Laughter Exercises

Acting and mime techniques; children's playgames.

Milkshake Laughter

"Pretend you are holding two imaginary glasses of milk. Pour one into the other,

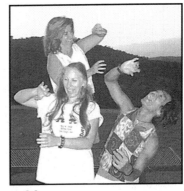

saying "Aee..." Pour the second into the first, saying (a little higher) "Aeee…" Then lean back, "drink" and howl. Look around and nod at the others, offer a toast - what a great milkshake you have - so do they!"

Appreciation Laughter

"Do gestures of appreciation: The tip of the index finger meets the tip of the thumb to make a small circle ("O-kay!"); use a "thumbs-up" gesture. Walk around

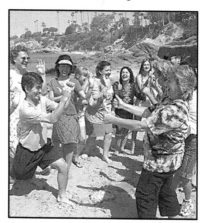

expressing appreciation (as if saying "Great job!" "Well done!" "Alright!" – but only laughing, no words). You can also applaud, throw kisses, 'Give me five,' etc. "

Motorbike Laughter

"Straddle your invisible motorbike. To start

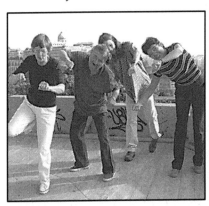

the engine it's going to take three times (turning the handle, pushing down one leg). First time: "*Ha*-ha-ha-ha-ha." Second time: "*HA*-ha-ha-ha-ha-ha." Then it starts up: "Ha-ha-ha-ha-ha..." Drive all around on your laugh-powered bike. Don't let gravity stop you; you can fly if you'd like!"

Category 3: Value-added Exercises

We take potentially stressful events and recondition ourselves to greet such events with lighthearted playfulness.

Argument Laughter ('Naughty-Naughty')

"Pretend to 'argue' by waggling your index fingers at each other. Playful only, nothing serious!"
(Follow with "Forgiveness", p. 111)

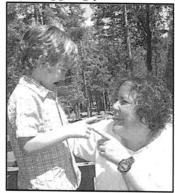

Credit Card Bill Laughter (Visa Bill)

"In the hands hold an imaginary bill" (or

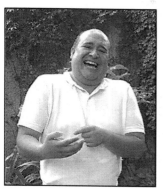

report card, or letter). "Open the hands, palms towards you. That which you see makes you laugh; show your palms and share with others."

Empty Pockets (No Money) Laughter

"Show your pockets to be empty. Laugh with

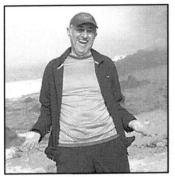

palms up. It doesn't really matter! Walk around and sympathize with others."

More Positive Effects of Laughter

Developing Emotional Intelligence (Emotional Resiliency)

The consistent practice of intentional laughter, especially "value-added" exercises as described above, allows us to experience emotions in a safe and pleasurable manner. In an environment free of judgment, we allow ourselves a wider range of feelings than we might otherwise find socially acceptable. Thus we expand our emotional range and develop our ability to handle any situation, secure in the knowledge that we can return to a state of happiness as soon as possible.

"God is a comedian, performing for an audience too afraid to laugh. " -- Voltaire

The stress/alarm response is appropriate only in response to a genuine life-threatening emergency. Once we can switch our reaction from stressful to playful, we will live healthier, less stress-filled lives. Practicing laughter deliberately will make it easier for us to laugh along with whatever life brings. To respond to the words of Voltaire: we learn to "laugh along with God". Besides: **"The sense of humor of God is weird**." -- Dr. Kataria

Don't Wait to Have a Happy Childhood

Laughter Yoga has us consciously and deliberately reconnect with the joy *which was our lifestyle* - hopefully - when we were children. A child may laugh hundreds of times per day (the *I Ching*, a Chinese book of philosophy, suggests that children laugh 200 times daily). Yet adults often laugh fifteen or fewer times per day. (Do you remember the last time you laughed even 100 times in one day? A good Laughter Yoga session can provide you with at least 100 bouts of legitimate laughter.)

The philosophy of Laughter Yoga affirms that the true potential of the human experience is to live in a state of Joy.

You now have easy access to that Joy. All you need do is: let go of seriousness, and laugh and play as if you were a carefree five-year-old child.

"It's never too late to have a happy childhood. Let's start right now!"

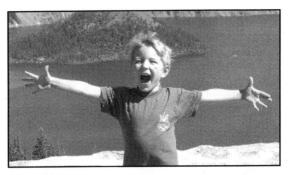

Hilarity Yields Creativity

Laughter Yoga also helps to balance the activity in the two hemispheres of the brain. During our waking hours we engage in mostly Left-Brain activity, characterized by comparing, analyzing, and predicting. But Laughter Yoga is largely a Right-Brain activity, characterized by playfulness, exuberant emotional expression and present-centered awareness.

By allowing the more vigorous activity of the right side of the brain, we provide a fertile breeding ground for creativity – seeing beyond previous restrictions and constructs, and imagining new, previously unimagined possibilities. This aspect of Laughter Yoga can be especially attractive to people whose careers make regular demands for new, creative ideas: designers, artists, composers, people in the fields of advertising and marketing, etc.

Pioneers of Emotional Health

Laughter Yoga might be said to be part of the Positive Psychology movement. Instead of focusing on negative trauma from the past as the source of our neuroses, we focus on positive elements; what we can do here and now to improve our life experience and enjoy living in the present.

Important predecessors of the Positive Psychology movement include the following innovators.

Dr. Benjamin Rush (1745–1813), sometimes 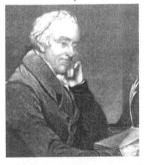 called "The Father of American Psychiatry", was one of the signers of the United States' Constitution. Dr. Rush suggested that when a person was having mental problems (e.g., lack of energy, or anxiety such that they could not function productively) they might be treated as having an illness, rather than as a criminal (engaged in a "crime" such as vagrancy). They needed help or counseling, not a prison sentence.

William James (1842–1910) theorized about the connection between emotions and the body: the mind-body link (see "Motion Creates Emotion" p. 91). He put forth the then-radical idea that by choosing a physical stance 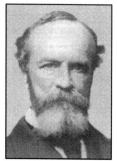 we could directly influence our emotional state. As James put it: "The greatest discovery of my generation is that a human being can alter his life by altering his attitudes of mind."

Swamis of Happiness – from Woodstock to Bombay

The 20th century also witnessed "Positive Thought" luminaries in the East (the Orient).

In the 1920s and 30s, when Swami Sivananda (1887-1963) noticed his yoga students taking life too seriously, he would instruct them to accompany him down to the riverside. "No more these gray faces," he would say. At the river's edge they would engage in humorous banter and joke-telling, enjoying abundant laughter.

Meher Baba (1894-1969) popularized the phrase "Don't worry, be happy" during the 1930s-1960s. He told his students worldwide to refrain from focusing on negative emotions like worry and fear, and instead focus on being happy and helpful to others.

Swami Satchidananda (1914-2002), most renowned during the 1950s-1970s, advised that all human beings have been provided with a Barometer of Truth; a way to determine if a proposed course of action is in one's Highest Good.

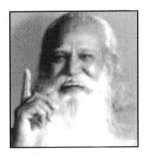

This measure of "rightness", a gift from the

Divine Intelligence which created us, is our feelings - more specifically, the feeling of happiness. If faced with an important decision ("Should I take that job? Should I marry that man?") Satchidananda instructed us to enter into a meditative state, pose the question, and listen for our feelings. If I react with feeling dread or terror, that suggests that the idea is not in my best interests. If I react with feelings of delightful anticipation, this may in fact be the best path for my spiritual well-being.

Satchidananda was the swami (teacher) who opened the Woodstock music festival in 1969. There were plenty of reasons why that Festival could have been a disaster from the start: There were far too many people, the toilets were not working, the hills had become rivers of mud – it could easily have been a miserable time for all. But the swami took the stage, sat peacefully, and had the audience members engage in Yogic breathing practices and gentle chanting. He encouraged everyone to focus not on the problems, but rather on the friendship and like-mindedness between them all. By encouraging everyone to take responsibility for their own feelings and make sure *everyone* had a good time, the festival was off to a great start. This event was reputed to be one of the most significant and joyful expressions of that generation.

Osho (1931-1990), earlier known as Baghwan Shri Rajneesh, offered his followers a practice called the Mystic Rose Meditation. Every day for one week, a group would get together and laugh for two hours. (Some of the participants might have their eyes closed or be blindfolded; unlike Laughter Yoga, there was no urging that they interact with each other playfully.) Next, every day for a week, the group would gather and cry for two hours. The next week, for two hours each day they would sit in silent meditation, witnessing their own thoughts and attempting to achieve perfect inner silence. This was said to be a life-transforming experience.

Western Science Weighs In on Laughter and Stress

Negative emotions/stress are bad for your health

Hans Selye (1907-1982) was a Hungarian research scientist who did his most significant work in Canada. Experimenting with mice, rats, and eventually 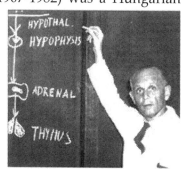 human beings, he examined the effects of stress on health.

Doctor Selye found that continued stressful, negative emotions - fear, anger, loneliness, resentment - had deleterious health effects. People who experienced constant anger often had heart problems; frequent worrying led to stomach ulcers; long-term grief or sadness suppressed the immune system.

Positive emotions/happiness are good *for your health*

Norman Cousins (1915-1990) was an American journalist, the publisher of the 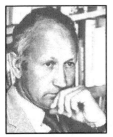 *Saturday Review of Books.* In 1968 during a peace-building mission to Russia he was unintentionally exposed to severe environmental toxins. Upon his return, he was diagnosed with Ankylosing Spondylitis, an auto-immune disorder.

Cousins' condition was so painful he said it felt as though he had been run over by a truck, and every bone in his body had been crushed. And that's how it felt all the time.

Cousins was told he had a 1-in-500 chance of survival. Some doctors estimated he had only six months to live. He was advised to clean up his affairs, say goodbye to his friends, and rest in the hospital, where he would receive pain-relieving medication for his last few months.

Instead of following their advice, Cousins checked *out* of the hospital and checked *in* to a comfortable hotel. Under the supervision of his physician, Cousins used himself as a guinea pig in an experiment on the potential benefits of positive emotions. (Cousins also received large doses of intravenous vitamin C.)

He was aware of the research by Doctor Selye (p. 49) which had shown the negative effects of emotional distress. Cousins hypothesized: if negative emotions are bad for health, perhaps positive emotions might be good for health.

He worked hard to have a positive attitude. He was supplied with a movie projector and numerous funny films – comedies by W.C. Fields, the Marx Brothers and others, as well as reruns of the television program *Candid Camera*. One of the first things Cousins noticed was that if he laughed for a good 10 minutes, he would experience relief from his pain.

"Ten minutes of genuine belly laughter had an anesthetic effect and would give me at least two hours of pain-free sleep."
-- Norman Cousins

The pain relief from laughing allowed him to obtain some much-needed rest. Frequently he would have a session where he would watch comedy films until he had 10 minutes of laughing; then the projector would be turned off. Two hours later, Cousins awoke to find the pain had returned. The projector would be turned on again and he would watch more amusing films, again seeking enough laughter for effective pain relief.

In six months, Cousins no longer suffered from Ankylosing Spondylitis. He later wrote an influential book on the topic of improving one's health through positive emotions: *Anatomy of an Illness – as Perceived by the Patient*. The book was on the New York Times Bestseller List for more than 40 weeks. Cousins became a lecturer at the UCLA School of Medicine, speaking on the topics of the deleterious effects of stress and the beneficial effects of positive emotions. He wrote several more books and helped to support solid research into improving health through healthy emotional states. Norman Cousins lived 20 years beyond his initial diagnosis as "terminal".

Research scientist Dr. Lee Berk was one of the beneficiaries of Norman Cousins' investment in having hard science validate the health benefits of laughter and positive emotions. Berk's research showed that 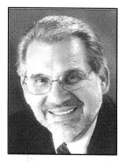 mirthful laughter can improve the functioning of the immune system, including natural anti-cancer cell activity. His fascinating explorations into "The Psychobiology of Hope" have shown that merely thinking positive emotions will have positive physiological effects in the present.

Dr. William Fry's research showed that

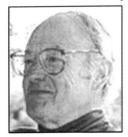 laughter had benefits similar to aerobic exercise – "Internal Jogging". Fry noted positive effects on the cardiovascular, respiratory, digestive, and eliminative systems. He also discussed the pain-relieving abilities of laughter, ascribing these effects to the production of Endorphins.

Dr. Hunter "Patch" Adams has taken laughter and joyful sharing to new heights. Well-versed in the psychopharmacology of positive emotions, Dr. Adams is a strong advocate for the healing power of humor, compassion, and interpersonal connection. Patch takes healthful emotions into the field.

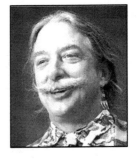

Participants in Dr. Adams' worldwide

clowning programs need no formal training. All they need do is slap on a red nose, open their hearts, and head into some of the most miserable places on Earth: refugee camps, places of extreme poverty, etc. There, by being open and childlike with others, the magic of connection and laughter occurs: faces light up, pain is relieved, and joy emerges. Patch offers his medical services at no charge.

The Kataria Breakthrough – 1995

The sciences of medicine – Physiology and Chemistry as well as Psychology – had shown that laughter is good for health. The challenge before the medical community was this: How can we produce laughter on demand? How can we give a prescription for a person to laugh, and be able to rely on that prescription being filled?

Watching funny movies or listening to recordings by comedians may not always work to elicit laughter. Once we've heard a joke for the first time we are not likely to laugh when we hear the same joke later. Some people may not find certain styles of humor amusing at all - the rapid-fire jokes of a Henny Youngman-type comedian might not prove laugh-provoking to an audience who prefers the sarcastic humor of Don Rickles. Some jokes might be found offensive, irrelevant, or even unintelligible.

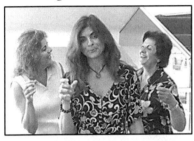

One audience may not understand jokes at all if they contain references to specific materials or cultural customs. (Do you know what a "burqa" is? Or a "buggywhip", or an "exhaust manifold"? If not, you probably would not understand a joke whose punchline involved such an item.)

A breakthrough in the application of laughter as a deliberate practice can be traced to a medical doctor from India, and his wife, a teacher of traditional Yoga.

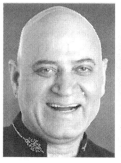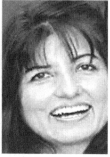

In 1995 Dr. Madan Kataria collaborated with his wife Madhuri to create a unique system whereby anyone can *dependably* laugh for a duration sufficient to obtain the benefits of therapeutic hilarity. The Laughter Yoga method has us laugh deliberately, as a form of exercise. The laughing occurs in a group. Thanks to personal interaction, good eye contact and childlike playfulness, laughter quickly becomes genuine.

"Laughter Yoga is the only technique that allows adults to achieve sustained, hearty laughter without involving cognitive thought. It bypasses the intellectual systems that [typically] act as a brake on laughter." -- Bill Gee, former Director of Laughter Yoga International

(A biography of Dr. Kataria appears on pp. 94-103)

The research of Professor Robert Provine 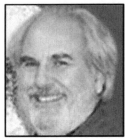 was elaborated in his book *Laughter – A Scientific Investigation* (2000). Instead of watching chimpanzees in their natural environment - the jungle, Provine's researchers spied on *human* subjects in *their* native environment - campus courtyards, shopping malls, lines waiting to get into theaters, etc.. This field research showed that people laughed as a result of hearing a joke only 18% of the time (less than one time out of five). 82% of the time (more than four times out of five) when one person laughed, the "trigger" which had resulted in the laughter response was *not* a joke, but rather was an expression of a social relationship; an offer of playfulness, stress release or other pleasurable shared experience.

"Laughter is not a result of jokes. Laughter is a form of communication." --Dr. Robert Provine.

Psychologist Steve Wilson is an accomplished lecturer and workshop leader in the field of humor to improve the workplace and one's personal life. In 1998 he traveled to India to give presentations on the 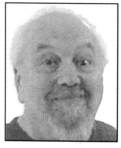 benefits of a humor-filled workplace. Wilson discovered Dr. Kataria and the "no-joke" Laughter Club phenomenon and was profoundly impressed. The following year, Wilson brought Dr. and Mrs. Kataria over to the USA for a "World Laughter Tour". After the Kataria's returned home to India, Wilson developed a version of practical therapeutic laughter. Wilson's "World Laughter Tour" has trained thousands of Certified Laughter Leaders. (A history of the first World Laughter Tour - which consisted of Dr. Kataria, psychologist Steve Wilson, and nurse Karyn Buxman - can be found in an article by the present author on Dr. Kataria's website: http://www.laughteryoga.org/blog/blog_detail/256 .)

Karyn Buxman, an award-winning speaker

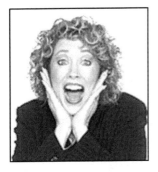

and nurse, has been a consistent champion of adding more laughter (and humor) to one's personal life and the workplace. A past president of the Association for Applied Therapeutic Humor (AATH), Nurse Buxman was part of the first USA tour with Dr. and Mrs. Kataria and Steve Wilson.

Patty Wooten, also a former president of AATH, is a practicing nurse and a renowned advocate of hospital clownery. Her excellent book *Compassionate Laughter* (1996) is an outstanding resource for the scientific validation and practical application of therapeutic laughter.

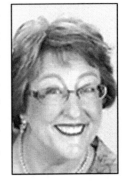

Attain "No-Mind" to Set Laughter Free

For nearly five decades research has shown the health potential of laughter. So why is it so hard to laugh, abundantly, and reliably?

Our "lack of facility to laugh" can be traced to a specific facet of our human experience: the Critical Mind, sometimes referred to as the Discerning or Judgmental Mind.

It's a good thing to have a Critical Mind. This Mind helps us remember our name, where we live, how to drive a car, which way to turn the key in the lock to our front door. It also reminds us, based on prior experiences, who we should trust and who we should avoid. But unfortunately it never rests, and when it comes to laughing, the Mind can be our worst enemy.

The Critical Mind stops us from laughing with the challenge: "Why *should* I laugh?". Mind requires that its standards be satisfied before it allows us the expression of laughing. The resulting laughter, when "approved", operates on a very Adult level.

Adult **Laughter** is:

* **Mental-based**

* **Highly Conditional** – triggers for laughter must satisfy several requirements, such as:

~ **May be Censored for Appropriateness** -"What will others think of me?" "How will I be judged if I laugh?" "Is it appropriate for me to laugh with *these* people?"

~ **Must be Perceived as New** - "I already heard that joke. I'm not laughing at it again.)

~ **Must Respect Values** - "I find that joke offensive. There is no way I will laugh at such humor."

~ **Must Make Sense** - operate within an understood language, use shared cultural references: "Voolay-voo coochay..."(?) "What *is* a 'Gecko', anyway?"

The solution to this problem - *The Kataria Breakthrough* - is to laugh with relative disregard for the Critical Mind. We "Laugh for No Reason" - more accurately: we laugh *Free* of Reason. We laugh deliberately, as a form of exercise.

"Laughter is too important to be dependent on jokes." -- Madan Kataria

This intentional laughter responds to the

Critical Mind's objection "Why should I laugh?" with the mind-befuddling answer: "Just laugh!" Just do it. Laugh for no reason. The health benefits follow anyway.

This *Mind-Free* **Laughter** is:

* **Body-based** - "Motion creates Emotion" (see Appendix, pp. 91-93); perform the physical expression of the emotion of happiness, and the physiological equivalent occurs

* **Relatively Unconditional**: playful and childlike

~ **Has us Laugh "with" (not "at") each other** - there is no judgment or criticism, no concern about "appropriateness"

~ **Has No Requirement for Novelty** or "Freshness" - with childlike playfulness, every moment is a delight

~ **Can be Nonsensical** - no need for shared language nor cultural values; laughers can share via nonsense talk, aka gibberish

Thanks to this innovation from a medical doctor and a yoga teacher, we can laugh at will for as long as we desire. We can produce laughter on demand, and need not remain victims of stress, ever again.

The Author's Story

I Was a Teenage Yogi-for-Fun

When Your Author was a teenager, two things happened which changed the course of my life. One was all about laughter. The other was all about Yoga.

COMEDY --- At the age of sixteen I began performing at the Renaissance Pleasure Faires, outdoor festivals in California which recreated an English country fair at the time of Shakespeare. Our comedy troupe *Cock & Feathers* offered mime, juggling, outrageous puns and slapstick comedy. We were often described as a Renaissance Marx Brothers act.

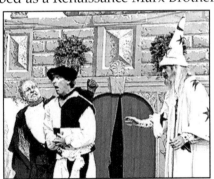

Cock & Feathers "Magical Mummery Madness"
(from left: Sandey Grinn; the Author; Billy Barrett)

Our shows were popular and influential, but despite the quality of our material and presentation, at times we failed to elicit laughter. As an entertainer there is always pressure to be funny, original, polished, etc. When you are attempting to get people to laugh but they are *not* laughing, this is called "dying onstage." This situation is, to use the vernacular of the time: "a Bummer."

YOGA --- Around the same time I became a student of traditional Hatha Yoga. My teacher was Swami Turiyananda of the Integral Yoga Institute of Santa Cruz. (The school of Yoga founded by Swami Satchidananda, pp. 46-48)

By age eighteen I was leading Yoga classes. I loved the health benefits and

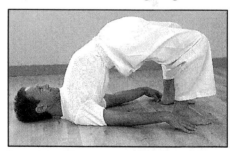

flexibility from my Yoga practice, but felt

something was missing. Yoga students generally keep to themselves, and I felt lonely from the lack of interpersonal connecting.

In 2003, one of my Yoga students told me about a park in India where 200 people gathered at six in the morning and laughed for an hour.

The 'comedian' side of me heard: "Laughing for an hour? How did they get people to laugh that much?"

My 'yoga teacher' side heard: "200 people gathering, at six in the morning – in India, the home of Yoga? What incredible dedication!"

I searched and happily found Dr. Kataria's School. In May 2005 I traveled to Switzerland and studied with Dr. and Mrs. Kataria.

I began laughing daily, gave Laughter Yoga seminars regularly, and started the Laguna Laughter Club (June 21, 2005), which initially met three mornings per week. In October a graduate of my first Leader Training, David Sullenger, offered to lead the club three additional mornings. Two months later we expanded to evening sessions on Saturday and thus became the first Laughter Club in the world outside India to meet seven days per week.

Since December 2005 the Laguna Laughter Club has met every day. At the time of writing, it remains the only club in the world outside Asia which meets seven days per week. Through April 2016 the club has welcomed 35,000 laughers in our eleven-year history of offering intentional hilarity by the sea, always free of charge.

* Comedians, take note: When guiding a Laughter Yoga session, there is no pressure to be an Entertainer. A Laughter Exercise Leader is not a performer; rather, they are a helpful Coach, assisting the participants to practice their own self-generated hilarity. And here's a bonus: at a Laughter Yoga session, each and every session, a participant *can* have the best laughs of their entire life. All they have to do is: be *willing* to have such a fabulous laugh. And then, *Do It!*

* Fellow Yogis, please be aware: In contrast to the social *isolation* typical of Yoga practice, Laughter Yoga is based in social *interaction*. We look into each other's eyes, see our inner child and play together like little kids at a public playground. We truly have "fun" *together*.

This kind of interactive laughing results in true feelings of friendship. Laughter Clubs which meet frequently tend to generate a community of caring, sharing, laughter-loving friends. A Laughter Club "family" may provide unconditional acceptance, support, and encouragement to personal happiness.

The Author coaching a hospital support group in Laughter-as-Exercise

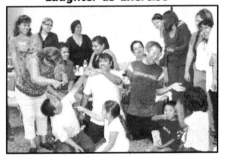

More Laughter Yoga Methods

Simulated Laughter + Integrating Technique: "Ho, ho, ha-ha-ha"

This is a combination of clapping, moving, and producing sound which offers many of laughter's benefits even if the participant is still thinking it isn't "real". The hand position is said to facilitate the flow of energy along the acupuncture meridians (energy pathways). Repetition provides an "anchoring" effect so participants can later evoke the Chemistry of Happiness without needing to laugh aloud.

Instruction:

"Place your hands so the palms and flats of the fingers will make contact. Clap your hands

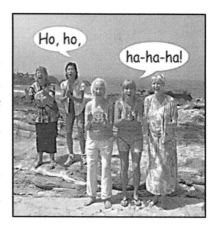

together in Cha-Cha rhythm: 'One, Two, One-Two-Three', making the sounds 'Ho, ho, ha-ha-ha!' Walk around, smiling and making good visual contact." (Everyone does simultaneously.) Perform frequently to conclude a laughter exercise.

Childlike Playfulness: "Very Good, Very Good, Yay!"

To achieve true contagious laughter we want to reconnect with our childlike sense of playfulness, and share this joy with our fellow laughers. A technique which can help us get in touch with the innocent joy of childhood is a combination of movement, clapping and verbalization we call "Very good, very good, Yay!"

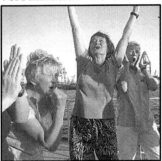

Instruction:
(Everyone does simultaneously.) "Clap your hands together once

while saying 'Very good'. Clap together again saying 'Very good'. Then extend and separate the arms with thumbs up," [or fingers wide apart] "saying 'Yay!'" Repeat three or more times - can be *many* more times. Perform frequently to conclude the practice of a laughter exercise.

The Power of Talking Nonsense: Applied Therapeutic Gibberish

During a laughter session participants are encouraged to laugh, abundantly and whenever they wish. But if they want to speak, only gibberish will do. Good meaningless gibberish allows for emotional expression and stimulates the Right- (intuitive) brain, while remaining relatively free of the Critical Mind.

To speak gibberish you can imagine talking like an infant ("Goo, goo, gaw-gaw gee gee"), speaking a language you don't actually know ("Tray bieeh, monn cwassa soojma"), or using popular nonsense phrases like "Blah blah blah" or "Yadda yadda bing

bing." (See the author's DVDs *Gibberish Sets You Free!* and *Gibberish Kit* - with Dr. Kataria, or the YouTube video "Gibberish 101".)

Gibberish can also be used as a trigger for laughter, as in the following exercise.

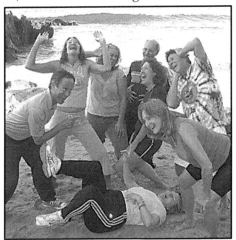

Gibberish Punchlines

Instruction:

"One person pretends to tell the last part of a joke – the punchline - but saying only a few words in gibberish. When they've finished, everyone laughs as if that was the funniest joke they'd ever heard."

Positive Affirmations

Near the end of a laughter session, the leader may run a segment where she makes statements declaring and reinforcing positive emotional states. After each statement, participants raise their arms in celebratory affirmation and shout out a childlike "Yay!" You do this even if you don't particularly "believe" the words of the affirmation; it's the emotion that counts, not the intellectual content. Positive affirmations might include: "We are the happiest people in the world!", "We are the healthiest people on the planet!", "We love to laugh!", "Life is good!", "We love our laughter club!", "We love everybody!"

Laughter Meditation

These are laughter techniques which have very little form or structure. A typical Laughter Exercise will often resemble a mime exercise: people are pretending to drink an invisible milkshake, ride an unseen motorbike, etc. In Laughter Meditation, there is no formal action to copy. We are a fountain of laughter, releasing our expression of joy; we open the faucet and let the laughter flow out.

By being so free of structure or form, Laughter Meditation can truly set us free from mental constraints. We can experience a spontaneity and freedom which may not be available through "copycat" laughing.

Laughter Yoga offers two distinct styles of Laughter Meditation:

1. *Sitting, with eyes open.* Participants seat themselves such that they can see one another. After the leader gives the command to start, they begin laughing in any way they wish, allowing the laughter to arise freely from within. The object is not to entertain others or to "make" them laugh, but rather to *allow* laughter to arise spontaneously, and enjoy the flow of contagious hilarity.

2. *Lying down, with eyes closed.* Participants lie on the floor and close their eyes. They cannot see each other, but they can hear one another. Upon the command to start, they allow laughter to flow out.

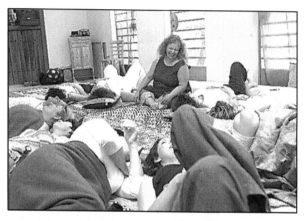

Many people consider the Laughter Meditation technique to be the highest expression of Laughter Yoga; the ultimate way to not only experience improvement to physical and psychological health, but also to realize laughter's most profound spiritual benefits.

Laughter Spirituality

The philosophy behind Laughter Yoga advises that there is more to us than our minds and bodies. We are in essence spiritual beings. Our true nature is to feel union with all: with our fellow humans, animals, the wind and trees, all of nature – the entire universe. "One With All That Is." When we are in the awareness of such unity, we will experience a constant state of blissful happiness.

The main challenge to the realization of our essential nature (and why we need to awaken to our inherent oneness with the universe) is the hindrance of our Critical Mind. This Critical Mind distances us from our fellow beings (p. 61). Mind is always comparing the way things are with the way the mind thinks they ought to be, so Mind sets up conditions which can make our lives miserable.

Laughter helps to dissolve the illusion of separateness. When we share our joyful hilarity with others, making eye contact and being playful, we tend to forget about our selfish problems and instead live thoroughly in the present moment. We see our laughter playmate as our brother/sister/friend, and the illusion of separateness between us fades.

The experience of laughter club members worldwide has shown that the regular practice of Laughter Yoga encourages spiritual values and lifestyle such as Kindness, Honesty, Compassion, Trust, Generosity, Forgiveness, Acceptance, Love, and Friendship.

Following are some of the author's preferred Laughter Exercises to encourage the realization of spiritual values:

Namaste Greeting (p. 34, 90), Appreciation (p. 37), Naughty-Naughty (p. 39), Forgiveness (p. 111), Credit Card Bill (p. 39), Empty Pockets (p. 40), Crying Laughter (p. 110), and Laughter Meditation (pp. 74-75),

(Readers may write to the author for the video of his conference presentation *The Spiritual Connection between Laughter Yoga and Classical Yoga.*)

Guided Relaxation

To achieve the maximum health benefits from a session of laughter, we need to include a period of rest. This can help to counterbalance the stimulation of intense laughter and play, and is essential to obtain all the potential physical benefits.

When we are in an active *Do, Do, Do!* behavior mode, our immune system is "on hold". We need to have a period of rest for it to recharge. Ideally, this restoration of immunity occurs when we sleep at night and take naps during the day, but often we don't sleep as much or as deeply as we would like to, and we don't take restful naps during the daytime. So we always want to include a time of relaxation after the exertion of a laughter session.

The session leader can guide the participants to mentally go over every part of their body, consciously directing that body part to relax. (Example: "Relax your toes. Release all tension or holding; let them go. The toes are relaxed. Now bring your attention to the soles of the feet. Release all tension in the soles of the feet. Allow the soles of the feet to relax..." Continue from the feet to the top of the head.) An effective guided relaxation may take five to twenty minutes.

Let there be Peace

Dr. Kataria, the creator of Laughter Yoga, has asked that laughter sessions end with a wish for world peace. (Instead of "wish" some people prefer a word like "intention", "prayer", or "visualization".) By aligning behind such a positive emotion, everyone can feel like they are making a contribution to the world family. We assert that we are laughing for a purpose higher than our own personal health; we are laughing for a healthier world.

Even if an individual is plagued by self-doubt, they can step outside of their own problems and express their support for a more joyful planet. Selfless positive reinforcement like this can boost one's self-esteem and improve our sense of worthiness.

A World of Enlightened Hearts

The technology of Laughter Yoga – unconditional, playful laughter, free of the constraints of humor – is spreading throughout planet Earth. Laughter "Clubs" (also known as Circles, Classes, Sessions, etc.) can be found by the thousands in more than ninety countries worldwide. You can find Laughter Yoga-focused conferences, conventions, and training programs on nearly every continent.

Laughter Yoga programs can be found in **schools and orphanages**. Children love the opportunity to laugh and be playful in class; teachers appreciate how laughter "breaks" can release the students' pent-up energy. Children 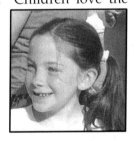 are then better able to focus and change gears - they can more easily move on to a new subject.

Laughter programs are becoming increasingly popular in mental health **clinics** and **hospitals**. Caregiver and other **support groups** are able to relieve the stress of their afflictions, and the pressures of giving care, and enjoy friendly interactions free of guilt.

Improving Quality of Life for Elders

Laughter programs are growing rapidly in the field of elder care. When an older person is moved to a care facility, they are often emotionally stressed. They've lost their home, their occupation, their autonomy, their family's proximity and their health. Now they find themself in an institution, surrounded by a lot of sick old people. There is a tendency to withdraw and isolate, which sets up the likelihood of becoming depressed.

Laughter Yoga is for everyone
Laughter Club at a Senior Center

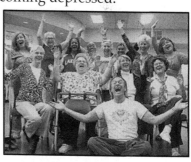

Laughter sessions can be lifesavers for elders in such a situation. By laughing, they have less anxiety and tension. Playful interaction makes boredom disappear. Participants feel more comfortable with one another, and caring friendships often develop naturally. Improved functioning of the immune system may result in better resistance to colds and infections.

Laughter in the World of Business: What if everybody *loved* going to work, every day?

In the workplace, regular laughter sessions have been shown to **increase job satisfaction** and boost employee **morale**. A more joyful work environment leads to **reduced employee turnover**; healthy laughing results in **healthier employees** and **less absenteeism**. The socializing aspect of Laughter Yoga improves **teamwork** and **cooperation**. The improved interaction between the Left and Right brain hemispheres leads to greater **creativity** and **innovation**.

Businesses in several countries start each work day with a laughter session. Management, staff, and rank-and-file workers all laugh together. Everyone starts the day in a genuinely cheerful mood, and this tends to last all day. These benefits are especially noteworthy in businesses where customers interact with the workers. Upbeat, happy workers lead to better customer relations. Employees of such businesses say they love going to work, each and every day, because they know that when they arrive they will have a wonderful time laughing with their buddies.

Laughter Yoga is well-received in **prisons**. Being incarcerated, inmates do not have much to laugh "at". Thus it is important that they learn to laugh "at" nothing. The Chemistry of Happiness is much enjoyed by the prisoners. Stress levels of guards and administrators are also lessened, whether they practice the laughter or only vicariously hear that the prison environment is experiencing joyful moments.

Luis Gomez is a Certified Laughter Yoga Teacher/Trainer who is regularly engaged by the governments of Mexico and Venezuela to bring laughter programs into prisons. Luis' slogan is *"Desencadena tu alegria"* - "Set Free your Happiness". Even if their bodies are stuck in jail, inmates can keep their spirits up by expressing unconditional childlike joyfulness. Attitude is improved by the laughter practice, and tensions are lessened throughout the facility.

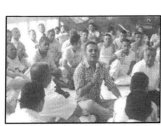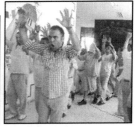

Luis Gomez guides prison inmates in Setting Their Happiness Free

Improving Sports Performance

Many activities require a balance between tension and relaxation. Too much stress or tightness can diminish effectiveness in sports like Golf, Tennis and Swimming. Some Laughter Yoga professionals give expert coaching for such sports. When the coach observes that the student is too nervous or tense, they'll order a Laughter Break. A few minutes of deliberate hilarity will relieve the tension; the student feels comfortable and relaxed again. Then the coach can work on the perfect balance between effort and relaxation to improve performance.

Laughter has been effectively combined with other like-minded exercise forms, including: traditional Hatha Yoga, T'ai Chi, Aikido and other Martial Arts, Expressive Dance, and Massage.

Benefits to Right/Left brain function make laughter a popular segment during Creativity Retreats. The world has seen Laughter Cruises, Laughter Tour Buses, Laughter Hikes… even Laughter Hayrides (and Laughter Sleighrides)! An extensive list of activities to which laughter can bring freshness and delight can be found at www.LYInstitute.org/Resources.

A Happier, Hilarity-Filled World
Laughing for World Peace

We have learned that positive emotions such as love, laughter and joyfulness improve health: physically, mentally, emotionally, socially and spiritually. We now know that people can laugh proactively, at will.

It is easiest to laugh if there are others present to laugh with. Laughter Yoga combines yogic breathing with laughter exercises in a context of childlike playfulness. By laughing *with* others - not "at" them - we can have abundant laughter, sufficient to assure ourselves of laughter's health benefits.

Laughter Clubs are flourishing all over the world. You can travel throughout our planet and by calling out "Ho Ho, ha ha-ha" or "Very Good, Very Good, Yay!" you will find yourself welcomed as a cherished friend into a family of Laughter Buddies. And these are people who only want to support each other in living lives filled with joy.

"People who are laughing together are generally not killing each other." -- Alan Alda

In the troubled nation-state of Israel, Laughter Yoga Teacher Alex Sternick brings together Arabs, Israelis and Iranians to laugh together for peace. Back home, these laughers' associates may tell them they should not associate with "the enemy". But Laughter Club participants know in their hearts that they would rather understand and enjoy the "others" instead of holding hate towards them.

Laughing together can heal emotional wounds. Children can laugh with their parents, grandparents, relatives; disabled persons can laugh with their caretakers. Anyone and everyone can laugh together, and through laughter new friendships result with ease. Sharing laughter leads to feelings of compassion, forgiveness, and caring - a sense of family; a family based in joy and trust.

Laughing with others promotes unconditional acceptance. When you can accept another person exactly as they are, and exactly as they are not; when you can look into their eyes and meet them in a place of pure joy and celebration, regardless of any appearances or circumstances; that kind of complete acceptance has another name: Love. This kind of Laughter *is* Love.

Share the Love

The world needs more friendship and joy, and Laughter Yoga is an effective system to fulfill that need. If you would like to be part of this worldwide 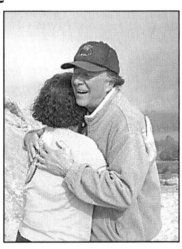 movement for health, joy, and world peace, please join us.

Visit a laughter club near you! The author's Laguna Laughter Club meets seven days per week on the sand in Laguna Beach, California USA. Go to **www.JoyfulB.com** to find Laughter Clubs worldwide.

Consider becoming a Certified Laughter Yoga Leader. In a two-day training program, you learn how to lead laughter exercises, start and operate your own Laughter Clubs, and bring more laughter into all areas of your life. Certified training can be found worldwide by contacting the author (web: www.LYInstitute.org; Email: Jeffrey@LaughterYoga.org), or through Laughter Yoga International headquarters in Bangalore, India.

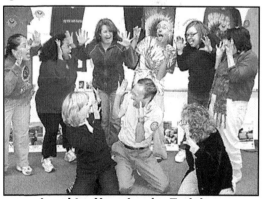

Laughter Yoga Leader Training
Irvine, California USA

Peace Be with You.

Laughing with another person, your heart and eyes open, your spirit as innocent as that of a five-year-old child, is an expression of sharing, honor and trust. Let us salute the laughter-light within each and every one of us.

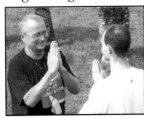 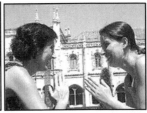

"*Namaste*. I honor the place in you where the entire universe resides. I honor the place within you of light, of love, of truth, of peace and of wisdom. I honor the place within you where, when you are in that place in you, and I am in that place in me, there is only one of us." -- Mohatma Gandhi

When you are in that place of light (-heartedness), and I am in that place, there is no separation between us. Then, we are One.

"Outside of concepts of right and wrong, there is a field. I'll meet you there." -- Rumi

'See you at the laughter playground.

-- Jeffrey Briar

Appendices

Motion Creates Emotion

Doctor Kataria refers to this concept as an inspiration behind the technique where we deliberately practice laughter to improve our physical and psychological health. This theory has its origins in the 19th century.

François Delsarte (1811-1871) was a French musician and actor who taught the art of emotional expression through gesture and voice. His work was based on observations of how people acted and reacted in real life. Delsarte proposed that emotional and physical expression are directly linked. He developed an acting technique that connected inner emotional experience with authentic human gestures.

The principles suggested by Delsarte were a profound influence on Modern Dance innovators Isadora Duncan (1877-1927), Ruth St. Denis (1879-1986) and Ted Shawn (1891-1972). A dancer's wish is not that their audience will be impressed with their footwork; rather, the performer's desire is that their Motion will elicit an Emotional reaction in their audience.

Fifty years after Delsarte's prime, psychologist **William James** (1842-1910) proposed that emotions were created *by* the body; that there was a direct link between a person's physical attitudes and their thoughts and feelings.

James suggested this experiment: Imagine a strong emotional reaction to some occurrence. Can you erase "its characteristic bodily symptoms"? Can you feel sadness without tears and drooping eyes; fear without a seizing of the breath and the urge to run way?

James said in such a case "We find we have nothing left behind, no 'mind stuff' out of which the emotion can be constituted." Emotions feel different from intellectual thoughts precisely *because* they have physical responses that give rise to internal sensations. Different emotions feel different from one another because they are accompanied by different bodily sensations.

James suggested that a person could undo a particular emotion by acting its opposite; by acting a certain way, we could cause ourselves to have specific emotional states.

Professional actors who portray the role of a depressed person have reported that after a prolonged period of time they begin to feel, in their personal life a similar negative emotional state. "Acting depressed" leaves them *feeling* depressed, even when their life circumstances do not merit this. It might take months to recover from such a role, until the actor feels "themself" again.

Depressed persons often have a hunched over body attitude and their breathing is shallow. If we imitate their body style, we can make ourselves feel weak and gloomy. In contrast, if we move our body in an uplifted way, we encourage uplifted feelings. An open-hearted body posture and energetic breathing will support us in feeling lively, enthusiastic and cheerful.

In the practice of Laughter Yoga, actions occur within the context of deliberate happiness. We gather for the express purpose of laughing and feeling good. We go through motions while consciously conjuring up the emotions of playfulness, joy and delight. We do the happy moves with accompanying gleeful laughter sounds, and happy feelings naturally follow.

The Kataria Story

Birth of a Consciousness
The Good Doctor, and Great Woman, behind the Laughter Movement

Madan Lal Kataria was born New Year's Eve, December 31, 1954 in the farming village of Mohrewala in Punjab, northern India (near the border with Pakistan). The homes of the village, huddled around cultivated fields, were built primarily from mud and cow dung. Mohrewala was not wired for electricity until 1971, when Madan was sixteen years old.

The village had a population of perhaps 200 souls. It was five miles to the nearest town, Firozpur. Daily life was full of hard work, but there were many simple pleasures. Younger children were always giggling and playing, and after a long day's toil neighbors would gather for singing, joking and storytelling. The sound of laughter often filled the air.

Madan's father was a farmer, as were almost all the inhabitants of Mohrewala. Tirath Ram Kataria had penetrating blue eyes and a thick moustache.

Madan described him as having a fiery personality, and easily angered - especially when money was lacking.

Madan's mother, Raj Karni, was attentive and affectionate. Madan credits her with teaching him the spirit of *Namaste* – to see the Divine God-essence in everyone he met. *Namaste* is a customary Hindu greeting, loosely translated as "The Divine within me honors the Divine within you".

Madan was the youngest of eight brothers and sisters. Mother Raj Karni had six other babies who did not survive childhood. Though both parents were illiterate, they observed that Madan was bright. They decided he should become educated. Raj Karni hoped that Madan, her youngest child, would someday become a medical doctor, and then return to care for the villagers. The nearest medical clinic was twenty-five miles away.

Mother Kataria sold her jewelry to pay for Madan's rooming in a hostel and for basic schooling in Firozpur. Madan, with his sister's help, was eventually admitted to the Government Medical College in the city of Amritsar.

Madan was a hardworking medical student who also excelled in theater, which he had studied since middle school. This knowledge of acting techniques served him well later when his therapeutic laughter technique called upon participants to "act happiness". In college he had to choose between his burgeoning theatre career or following his medical studies. Apparently, the world needed a Laughter Avatar more than another tall, handsome Bollywood star. Madan's decision was to pursue a career in medicine.

Upon graduation, Kataria moved to Bombay (Mumbai) where he not only secured a residency at the Jaslok Hospital and Research Center (at the age of 26) but he could also attempt to seek fame in Bollywood. Bombay was the heart of India's huge film industry. "I dreamed of becoming a rich and famous doctor," he recalled.

After completing his residency in 1986 Madan married Madhuri Sajnani, the daughter of a socially prominent police official from Rajasthan. Madhuri was a junior executive with Mahindra & Mahindra, a large automotive manufacturer based in Bombay, until 1993. A few years into the marriage, Madhuri studied classical Yoga at the Yoga Institute Santa Cruz West in Bombay, graduating in 1990. The Kataria's would often practice Yoga together.

In 1988, the same Year Madhuri began her Yoga studies, Doctor Kataria opened a general medical practice in Bombay in a respectable apartment block named the Lokhandwala Complex. His desire for greater fame and fortune led him to a number of ambitious enterprises. He bought a van and created one of the city's first mobile clinics. (This project flourished for four years – one of Dr. Kataria's few early successes.) He planned to open a chain of pharmaceutical companies, and a chain of private hospitals. He developed a series of First Aid Kits and a medical steam inhaler. All of these enterprises did not prove financially workable, and this eventually led to tension at home and with his family. His mother came to visit and noted that her youngest boy seemed stressed and unhappy. Back in the village he had been so inclined to laughter and playfulness. Why not return to Mohrewala and become the village doctor? "Give me two more years," Doctor Madan told his mom. He'd either make it in Bombay, or return to the village of his birth.

In 1991 Kataria started publishing the magazine *My Doctor*. Designed for the layperson, the periodical had articles on both traditional (Western) and alternative (Eastern) forms of medicine. The magazine used the symbol of an apple, as in the slogan "An Apple a Day Keeps the Doctor Away". At its peak, *My Doctor* had a circulation of 19,000 copies, with editions in both English and Hindi.

In his medical practice Kataria sometimes observed that when patients experienced periods of laughter, their conditions improved, regardless of the specific condition. One patient, with allergies, may have recounted that he had a visit from family and laughed for hours with his cousins; the doctor noted the man's allergic symptoms were improved. Another patient, suffering from recurrent depression, might have shared that he had gone to a festive celebration, laughed heartily, and his depression was relieved. Kataria decided to seek out the solid science confirming laughter's contribution to physical health.

Researching an article he planned to publish in *My Doctor* magazine to be entitled "Laughter – The Best Medicine" Kataria was particularly impressed with Norman Cousins' book *Anatomy of an Illness*, as well as the research of Dr. Lee Berk, which showed considerable health benefits from laughing.

One day - March 13, 1995 - at four o'clock in the morning, Kataria was struck by an illuminating idea. "If laughter is so good, why not start a Laughter Club?" People were already going to Bicycling and Jogging Clubs to improve their physical stamina, to Book Clubs to improve their literary skills, to Chess Clubs to improve their strategic thinking... why not a *Laughter* Club, to improve their health by practicing hilarity?

Dr. Kataria was so excited with his new idea he could hardly wait until 7:00 a.m. when he went to a local public park and began inviting people to join him to laugh deliberately to improve their health.

At first he was greeted with skepticism. "What, are you crazy?" his neighbors replied to his invitation. "This is India, we don't do such things." "No one would laugh out loud in a public park." Kataria asked over 200 people (a number equivalent to the entire population of his home village of Mohrewala!) but only four others joined him at the first laughter session, one of whom was his dear and only wife Madhuri.

At first, not knowing what else to do to evoke laughter, the group members stood in a circle; one person placed themself in the center and told jokes. The sound of their laughter was so attractive, within a week fifty people were attending the group. Newcomers were encouraged to return – and bring fresh jokes and funny stories to share.

"After about ten days, the stock of good jokes ran out," Kataria related. People started telling jokes that had been told earlier which, lacking novelty, did not elicit laughter. Some told jokes which offended others' religions, or were violent, or sexually vulgar.

A few women were attending, and they expressed their disdain: "Better to stop this laughter club than continue with such offensive material."

"No, no; laughter is too good," Kataria replied. "Come back tomorrow; I will come up with a way where we can laugh without using jokes." The

Laughter Club members departed for the day, intrigued with the idea of returning next time to laugh without jokes.

Kataria went home, baffled. He wondered: "How can people laugh if we don't have jokes or funny stories to laugh at?" He returned to the research on laughter and found treasure in the book "Emotions and Health," a collection of articles compiled by Prevention magazine. *

He read that even if laughter was fake – if a person was only pretending to laugh – the body made no distinction. The literature declared: by going through the *motions* of laughing, beneficial *emotional* and *physiological* changes *would occur* (see "Motion Creates Emotion" p. 91). Laughter itself, practiced as deliberate exercise, offered positive impacts on health, even without the comedy component.

"No problem," Kataria thought. "We'll just do pretend laughter." He breathed a sigh of relief.

He returned to the Laughter Club in the morning and shared the results of his research. Since the purpose of their gathering was to engage in laughter in order to improve their physical health -

not to learn new jokes to stimulate their intellect - they would start by doing "pretend" laughter. So he called for the first minute of Laughing for No Reason. "Are you ready? Start!"

At first, the participants laughed only mechanically. However, as they already felt comfortable being with each other, they looked around and saw one another laughing. Soon, their laughter shifted from "fake" to incredulous. Inside, they were thinking: "Why am I laughing? Why are *you* laughing?" "I don't know – we just *are*. And doesn't it feel great?! Ha ha ha ha ha!"

For many, the laughter became downright hilarious. People were falling to the ground, hysterical, tears of joy streaming from their eyes. Kataria recalled: "We laughed more that first day without jokes then we had laughed the entire two weeks up to that time."

The laughter had become real and contagious. The laughers were interacting playfully and were feeling fresh and energetic like young children.

Laughter Exercises were soon devised which were simple expressions of daily life: pouring the ingredients to make a milkshake, measuring a yard of fabric, performing household chores. These unpretentious, insignificant movements were now infused with deliberate hilarity. Madhuri contributed many exercises, some adapted from Yoga postures and breathing techniques, as well as developing the use of nonsense talking (gibberish) to reduce inhibitions and get laughter flowing.

Thus was laughter set free from the Critical Mind's demand to be appeased with jokes or humor. Instead of laughing "at" something perceived as *funny*, people were laughing "with" each other - while *having fun*.

"As far as your health is concerned,
laughter from having fun
is just as good
as laughing at something funny." -- Jeffrey Briar

* Kataria's treasured book was *The Complete Guide to Your Emotions & Your Health* by Emrika Padus (1986, Rodale Press, Emmaus, Pennsylvania).

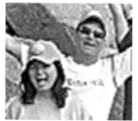

Dr. and Mrs. Kataria visiting Laguna Laughter Club in California (2006)

Contraindications

There are a few conditions which might make it inadvisable to practice hearty laughter. Laughter is a form of mild aerobic exercise and can involve a rise in inter-abdominal pressure, so it may be contraindicated if a person is suffering from any of these conditions:

- Recent Abdominal or Chest Surgery - you don't want to laugh your stitches open
- Hernia, Hemorrhoids - because of increased abdominal pressure
- Epilepsy - if the laughter is done in a regular, predictable rhythm, this might result in brainwave entertainment which could lead to an epileptic episode
- Late-stage Pregnancy - pregnant women can be advised to only laugh gently, in the throat and head
- Potentially contagious Respiratory Diseases such as cough, cold, flu, TB - this is primarily out of consideration for the other laughers present, that they would not be exposed to any potential contagion. A person with a mild cold or flu could certainly laugh gently by herself.

The Laughter Exercise Session

Formats for Laughter Sessions vary worldwide, but in general we always want to have: a warm-up; 15 to 20 minutes of Laughter; a period of Relaxation; and a wish for Peace. "Choosing Exercises" (p. 121) suggests the contents for some typical Laughter Exercise session.

1. Welcome: Participants are advised:

a) They are to Take Care of Themselves and experience No New Pain (p. 30). They can always modify any practice to fit their comfort level, or sit it out.

b) Everyone is to refrain from talking (speaking words in any real language) for the duration of the laughter segment. Speaking in "real words" invariably involves the Critical Mind (see p. 61) and during the laughter segment we want to be as free as possible from criticizing thoughts. Only the exercise Leader speaks during the laughter portion; participants are encouraged to laugh as much as desired (or to talk exclusively in gibberish/nonsense talk – pp. 71-72).

2. **Body Warm-Up**: We prepare for expressing ourselves with an all-over physical warm-up lasting three to ten minutes, composed of easy stretches and gentle vocalizations. (A video showing a simple five-minute warm-up can be seen on the author's website at www.LYInstitute.org.)

3. **Breathing Exercises**: Do one or two, then repeat the same Breathing Exercise(s) with laughter on the exhalation. (See pp. 19-20, 36, 115-117.)

4. **Laughter Exercises** (fifteen to twenty minutes):

Greeting (Namaste (p. 34) &/or Handshake); "Ho, ho, ha-ha-ha";

Two Exercises (pp. 34-40, 108-114, etc.) ending each with "Ho, Ho, ha-ha-ha" (p. 69);

One Exercise; "Very Good, Very Good, Yay!" (p. 70-71);

One Exercise; then an easy Stretch or Breathing exercise;

Six to eight more Laughter Exercises, interspersed with "Very Good, Very Good, Yay!," "Ho, ho, ha-ha-ha," and other easy Stretches/Breathing exercises.

5. **Positive Affirmations:** The Leader expresses a declaration like "We are the healthiest people in the world!" and the others respond with a vigorous cheer: "Yay!" (p. 73) The Leader says two or more additional affirmations (e.g., "We are the happiest people in the world!" "We love to laugh!" "We are having fun!" "We love everybody!" etc.), each followed by the group "Yay!" cheer.

6. **Laughter Meditation** (pp. 73-75)

7. **Guided Relaxation** (pp. 78-79)

8. **Wish for Peace; Announcements**

Laughter Exercises (a Happy Handful)

Here are simple activities to bring you more joy, new friends, and better health; laugh-evoking practices for any declared "playtime" for people of all ages. More fun than a pile of puppies, as much joy as finding buried pirate treasure... such are the delights you'll find from these cheerful practices.

All exercises are performed *while laughing.* No real words are spoken, except by the Leader while giving instructions. The word-examples given below are presented to indicate the feeling being expressed, but participants do not actually speak; they only make laughter sounds, or speak in gibberish. Laughers are encouraged to participate only at the level which feels comfortable for them.

The images were originally used with the Laughter Exercise Photo Flash Cards. You can order files to make these cards via www.laughter-exercise-cards.info. The website has translations of the exercise instructions into several languages. These pictures depict international laughter-lovers from twenty-three countries. These exercises, and many more, are in the book *The Great Big Anthology of Laughter Exercises* from the same author.

American Cowboy

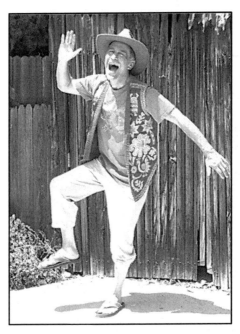

A Playful Exercise.

"Slap your thighs, one or both, like a cowboy from the Wild West: 'Yee-haw!' Raise up your big ten-gallon hat ('Howdy, Ma'm'); place the fists on the hips; ride a horse; lasso a steer and wrestle it to the ground; twirl your six-shooter guns. Use big, broad, roaring laughs, 'Hardy har har!'"

Calcutta Laughter

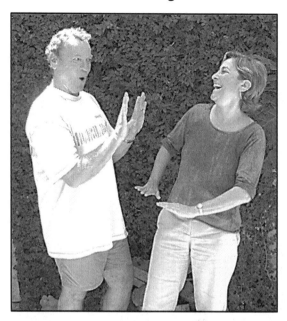

A Yoga-based exercise (variant of *Kapalbhati*, Skull-Shining Breath)

"Have your hands in front. Do two short sharp repetitions of 'Ho, Ho' with hands pushing forward; follow with two repetitions of 'Ha, Ha' with hands facing down and push sharply downwards. Include a slight bounce in the knees. You can do dance-like movements, hands to one side, above the head, etc. You can speed up."

Crying Laughter

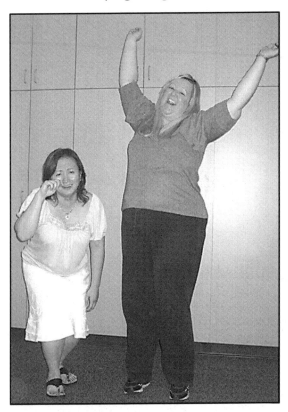

A Value-added Exercise.

"Cry while sliding down to a crouch; then happily laugh your way up. Repeat several times."

Forgiveness

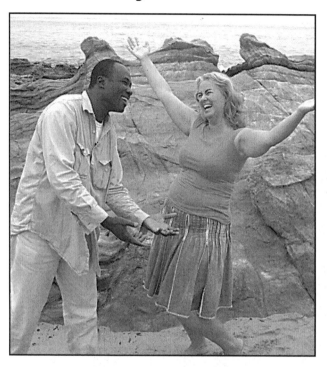

A Value-added Exercise.

"Do a gesture that indicates that you offer forgiveness, the arms apart and palms open. Apologize and 'ask' forgiveness of others. Forgive yourself, forgive everyone and everything."

Gradient Laughter

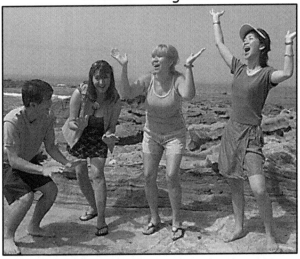

A Playful Exercise.

"Start with a smile, let it grow to a gentle giggle; allow to slowly build, (in vigor and volume, until roaring. Then let it gradually diminish back to gentle." (Everyone does together.)

Variation (following the exercise leader): "When I place my hands low, we laugh slow and gentle, like 'Ho… ho… ho, ho; ho…' When my hands are at shoulder height, we do moderate laughs: 'Ha-ha-ha-ha-ha.' When the arms are overhead, hilarious howling: 'Ho, hahaha, HEE Hoo-Hoo-Hoo-Hoo-Hoo!!' Follow along now…"

Laugh for No Reason

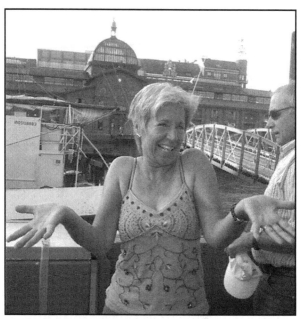

A Value-added Exercise.

"As if a passerby has just asked, 'Why are you all laughing?', turn the palms of the hands up, the elbows bent, shrug the shoulders, tap the forehead… as if to say 'I can't tell you why. We're just - laughing, for no reason!'"

One Meter

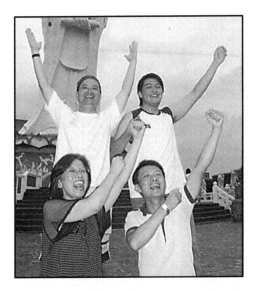

A Playful Exercise.

"As if measuring a length of cloth, start with the arms up to one side, the hands close together. Move one arm along the front of the body, as if measuring: 1) to the other arm's elbow, saying 'Aee.' 2) to that arm's shoulder joint, saying (a little higher) 'Aee.' Then 3) to the other shoulder joint; then bring the arms wide apart, the head slightly back; celebrate having succeeded in measuring a meter. Look around at the others – they've succeeded, too! We all did it, Yay!"

Breathing Exercises

Based in Yoga breathing (*Pranayama*) practices.

Arms Up The Front

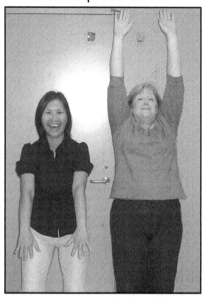

"Deeply inhale while bringing the two arms up above the head, the palms facing forward. Exhale fully while lowering the arms down to the thighs."

To make a Laughter Exercise: "Laugh while lowering the arms. You can walk around, and continue laughing as you raise and lower the arms at will."   (Also on pp. 19-20.)

Hastasana (Palms Together Above Head)

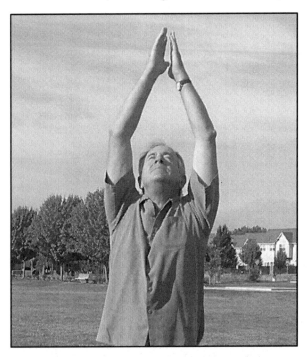

"To prepare, bring your palms together above the head with the arms straight. Inhale fully; then exhale completely, keeping the arms up."

As a Laughter Exercise: "While exhaling, walk around (arms remaining above the head with palms together) as you nod, smile and laugh, making eye contact with others. "

Butterfly Wings

(Angel Wings, "Montalbanasana", Reverse Prayer)

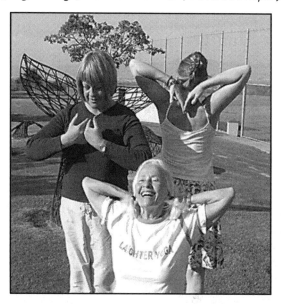

"Place the backs of your fingers together, then bring the arms up and behind the head. Your hands reach for the level of the shoulder blades. Inhale fully, stretching the elbows wide apart. Keep the arms where they are as you exhale completely. "

As a Laughter Exercise: "On the exhale, walk around, arms up and behind the head; laugh, nod, and smile while connecting with others."

How to Lead a Laughter Exercise

All sessions begin with the notification that students can participate at whatever energy level they wish ("Take good care of yourself" or "No new pain") (p. 30). Participants can modify any practice to suit their personal comfort level, or refrain from performing any activity which they think might cause them discomfort.

The Three "D's": *Declare, Demonstrate, Do*

Step 1: *Declare* (Denote/De-name). Give the name of the exercise.

"The next exercise is called 'Penguin Laughter.'"

Step 2: *Demonstrate*. Show physically how to perform the exercise, while simultaneously verbalizing the instruction.

"Start with your feet turned out [*place your own feet in this position:*], arms straight down by your sides, hands flexed, palms facing the floor. Walk around like a penguin [*do a stiff-legged walk, the upward-flexed hands swinging into and then away from the legs*]. Play with or follow behind the other penguins, laughing all the while [*make eye contact with other participants, lean towards them in greeting*]."

Step 3: *Do*. First: stop the demonstration. Then: give a clear "Command to Start." This is done with a sense of building up tension such that everyone will release into laughing together, all at the same time, the moment you give them the cue to do so.

"Okay, got your feet turned out? Ready --- set: *Go!*" (immediately burst into laughter). Or: "Penguins, are you ready? *Take off!*" Or: "Here we go: One, two, three, *Waddle!*"

Allow the exercise to run for *at least* fifteen to forty-five seconds. Some enthusiastic groups may run an entire minute or longer. Tune in to your team. Allow for space wherein participants can go beyond their initial effort, to explore nuances and get creative.

Conclude the exercise by calling out words of praise (like "Great job, everyone!" or "Fantastic!") or doing the "Ho, ho, ha-ha-ha" exercise (p. 69) or "Very good, very good, Yay!" (p 70) technique. To develop expertise in leading Laughter Exercises, see *The Great Big Anthology of Laughter Exercises* by the same author. Even better, attend a two-day Certified Laughter Yoga Leader training program (p. 89).

Choosing Exercises for Your Group

Select practices to best suit the abilities and needs of the participants. You might select vigorous exercises for a room full of energetic eight-year-olds, but gentler ones for a group of wheelchair-bound seniors.

Be considerate of any physical limitations. Elders often do not like to get down on the floor, as they may find it difficult to get back up. Sports-lovers and children may require physically challenging activities to avoid boredom. For starters, choose exercises that relate to the participants' real lives: people in business enjoy Cellphone and Jackpot; athletic folks like to laugh with sports victories; most adults relate well to Credit Card Bill (you can rename it "Report Card" for school-age children).

After a few sessions, when they trust your leadership and feel comfortable with one another, you can probably expand into any and all Laughter Exercises. Yes, you *can* have your stuffed-shirt business colleagues go to the Playground, stick out their tongues like Lions, and waddle around like Penguins. Above all: have fun - and share it!

120

Laughter Exercises suggested for specific groups:

Children under 13: Lion, Penguin, Bird, Playground, Naughty-Naughty, One-Word Gibberish Punchlines, Hot Soup, Shy, Hearty, American Cowboy, Appreciation.

Well-Dressed Ladies: Cellphone, Laughter Cream, Royal, Appreciation, Milkshake, Naughty-Naughty, Shy, Let Your Light Shine, Laugh at Yourself, Forgiveness, Silent, Gibberish Punchlines 2 "Quips".

Serious Adults (business professionals): Handshake, One Meter, Cellphone, Milkshake, Credit Card Bill, Jackpot, Motorbike, Gibberish Punchlines, Silent, Hearty.

Seniors: Royal, Laughter Cream, Appreciation, Milkshake, Cellphone (Telephone), Laughter Center, Laugh at Yourself, Vowels.

Find these and hundreds more in *The Great Big Anthology of Laughter Exercises*.

About the Author

When he was a child, Jeffrey Briar made funny faces for people to laugh at.

Nowadays, he teaches people how to laugh at absolutely nothing.

Since a teenager, he has played piano accompaniment for silent movie comedies, performed onstage in the most popular humorous act in the history of the Renaissance Pleasure Faires, and appeared on stage and screen as a lookalike for Charlie Chaplin, Stan Laurel and other comedy immortals. Simultaneously, he had a bustling career as a teacher of classical Hatha Yoga, conducting up to thirty sessions per week.

In 2005 he became a Laughter Yoga Teacher under the tutelage of Dr. and Mrs. Madan Kataria, the creators of this therapeutic laughter technique. Briar promptly founded a Laughter Yoga Club. The Laguna Laughter Club soon became the first club in the western world to meet seven days per week, and has welcomed 35,000 laughers.

Mr. Briar has produced numerous Laughter Yoga instructional videos (most with original musical scores composed by Mr. Briar) as well as audio CDs, instructional aids, and textbooks, including *Laughter Revolutionaries: Making the World Safe for Hilarity* and *The Great Big Anthology of Laughter Exercises*.

As a Laughter Yoga champion, Jeffrey Briar appeared on *CNN-TV with Dr. Sanjay Gupta*, *The Oprah Winfrey Show*, and *Dancing with the Stars*.

Jeffrey leads laughter exercises regularly at his social Laughter Club, at senior centers, for business presentations, and wherever he is needed. Having led and laughed every day for more than eleven years, Jeffrey Briar is probably the most experienced leader of Laughter Yoga exercises in the western world.

In 2011 he was appointed a Master Trainer for Dr. Kataria's Laughter Yoga International University. Currently, Jeffrey travels throughout the world sharing this unique technique whereby everyone can experience the benefits of hearty laughter without needing comedy or jokes.

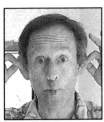
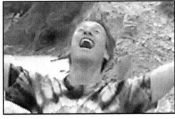

The Laughter Yoga Book
Compact Edition

Jeffrey Briar

www.LYInstitute.org
Jeffrey@LaughterYoga.org
1 (949) 376-1939

ISBN-13: 978-1478292135
ISBN-10: 147829213X

Made in the USA
San Bernardino, CA
18 July 2020

75622632R00071